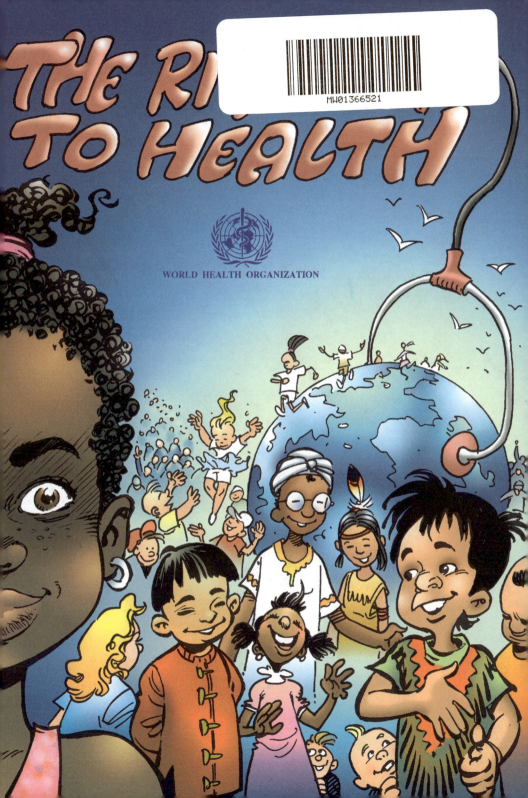

DRAW YOUR FAMILY

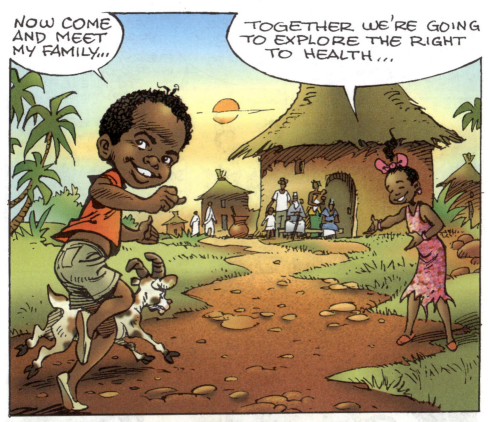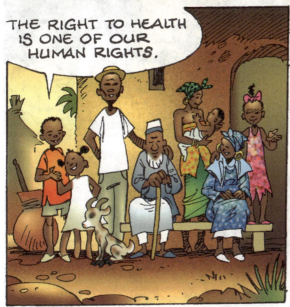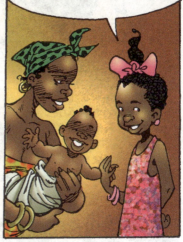

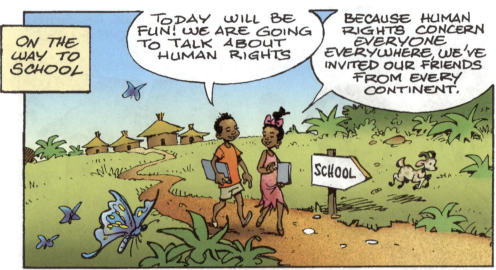
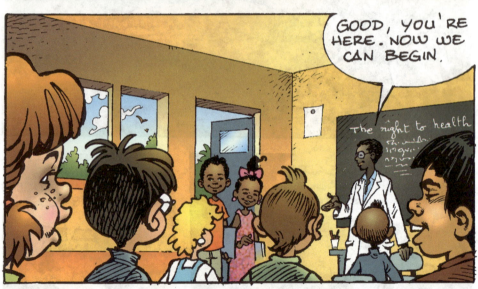
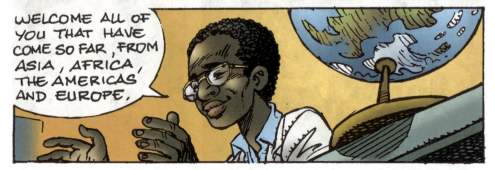

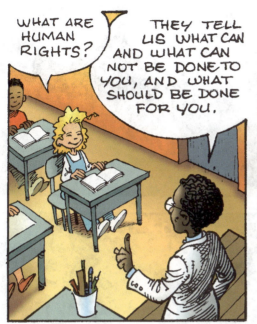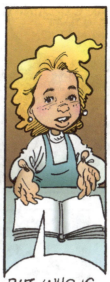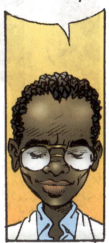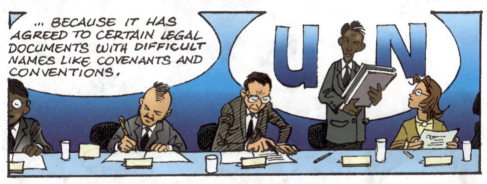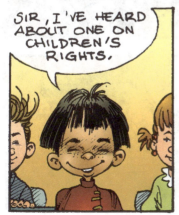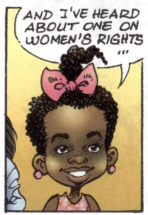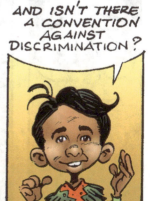

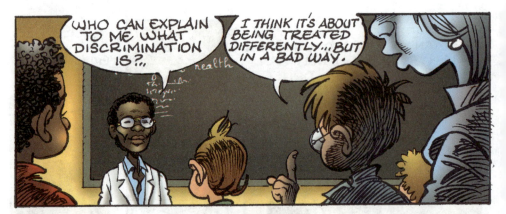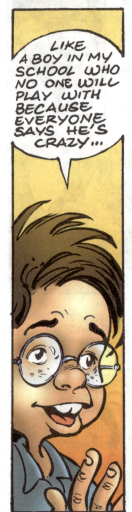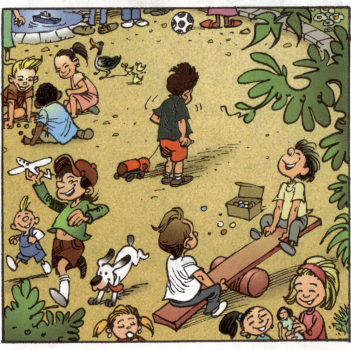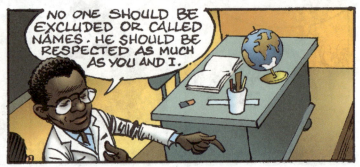

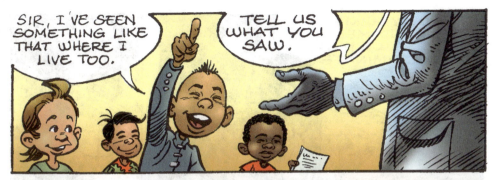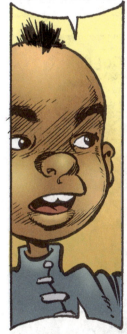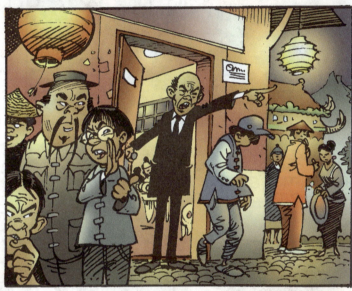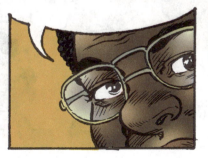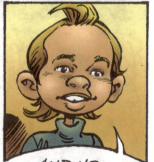

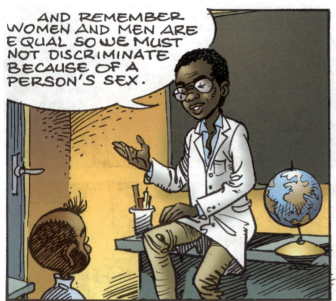
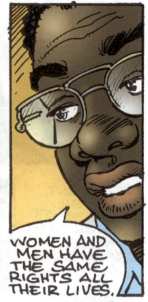
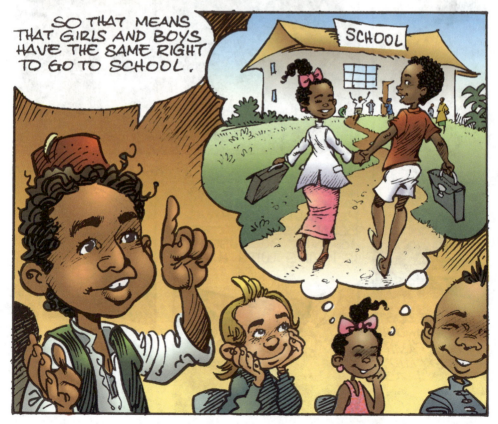

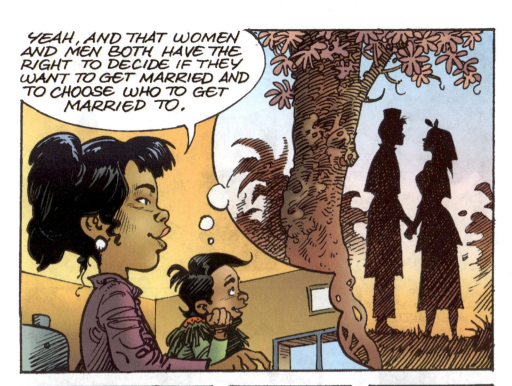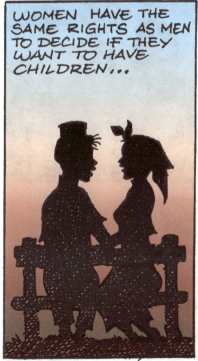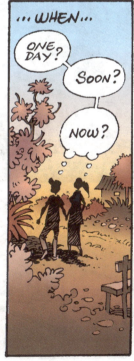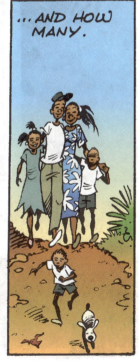

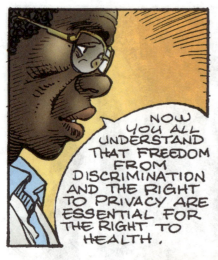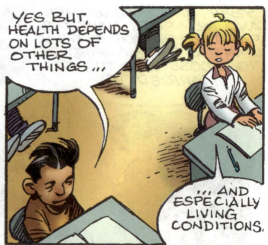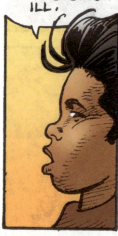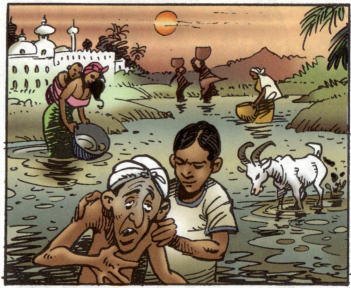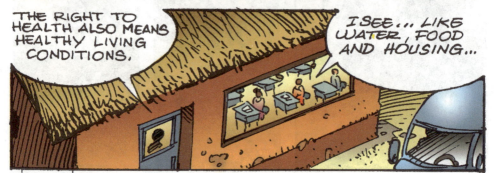

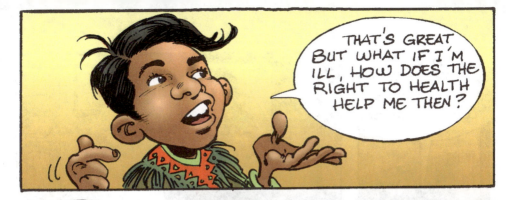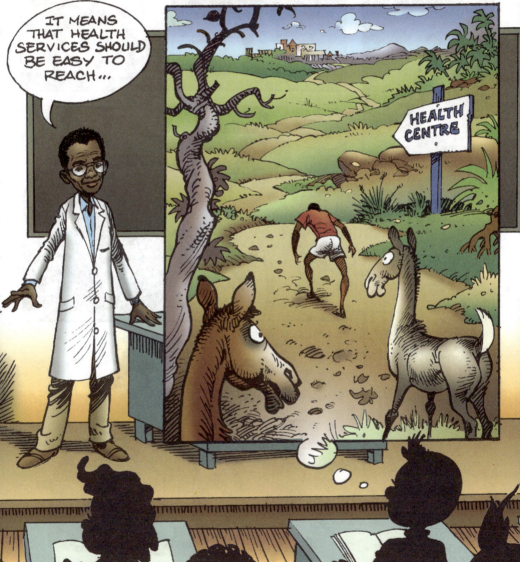

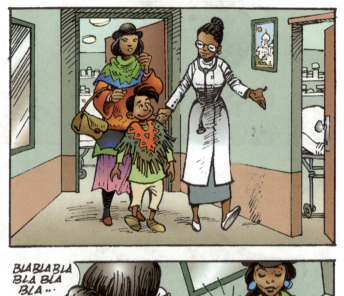

"...AND THAT WHERE YOU ARE CARED FOR YOU SHOULD BE TREATED WITH RESPECT."

"BLA BLA BLA BLA BLA BLA..."

"DON'T FORGET THAT YOU CAN ASK QUESTIONS AND EXPECT AN ANSWER..."

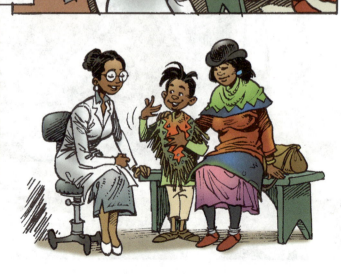

"YOU SHOULD BE LISTENED TO BECAUSE IT IS WHAT IS BEST FOR YOU THAT COUNTS."

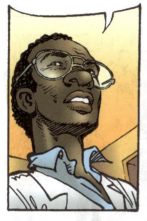
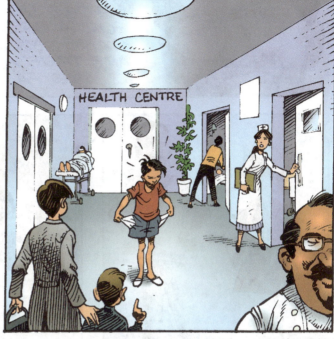
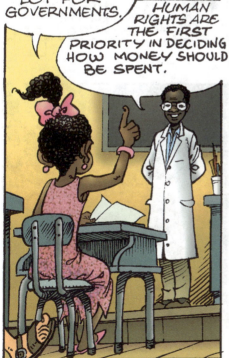
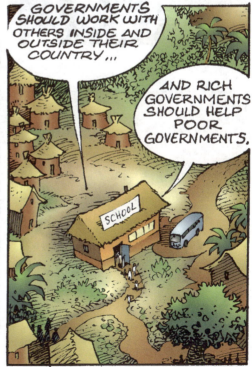

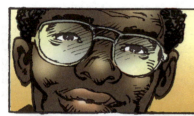

Before you go out for a break try this game: mark which boxes are true and which are false.

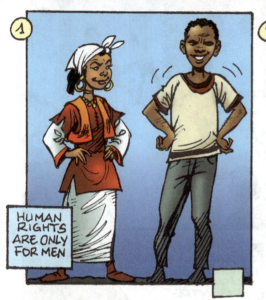

1. Human rights are only for men.

2. Human rights are for everyone... without discrimination.

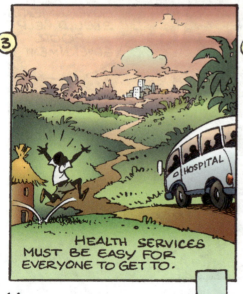

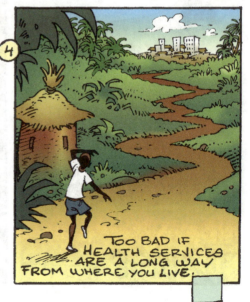

3. Health services must be easy for everyone to get to.

4. Too bad if health services are a long way from where you live.

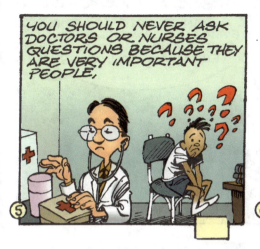
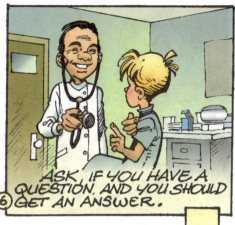
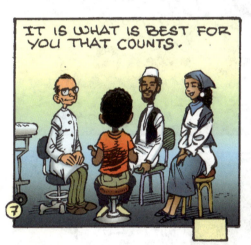
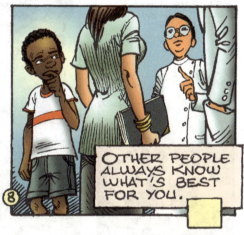
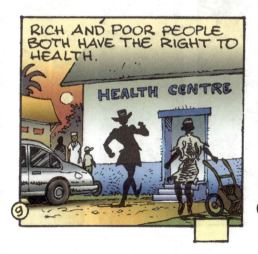
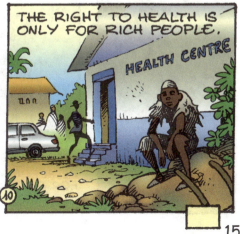

HAVE FUN OUTSIDE ON YOUR BREAK, BUT REMEMBER...

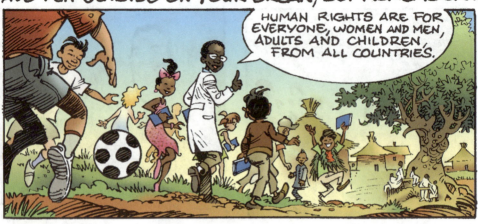

HUMAN RIGHTS ARE FOR EVERYONE, WOMEN AND MEN, ADULTS AND CHILDREN, FROM ALL COUNTRIES.

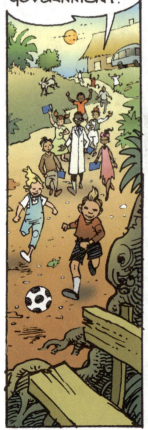

HUMAN RIGHTS ARE THE FIRST RESPONSIBILITY OF YOUR GOVERNMENT.

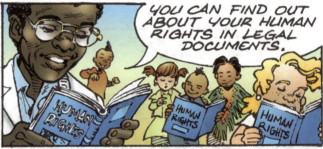

YOU CAN FIND OUT ABOUT YOUR HUMAN RIGHTS IN LEGAL DOCUMENTS.

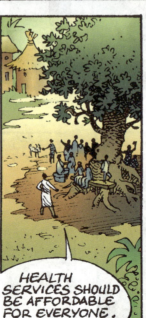

HEALTH SERVICES SHOULD BE AFFORDABLE FOR EVERYONE.

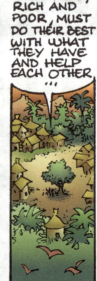

GOVERNMENTS FROM ALL COUNTRIES, RICH AND POOR, MUST DO THEIR BEST WITH WHAT THEY HAVE AND HELP EACH OTHER...

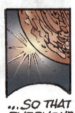

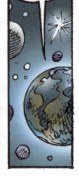

...SO THAT EVERYONE CAN ENJOY HUMAN RIGHTS.